Growing Gareth

Playing with two switches

Created by Luke Thompson

Co-author Caroline Bennett

Illustrated by Kat Willott

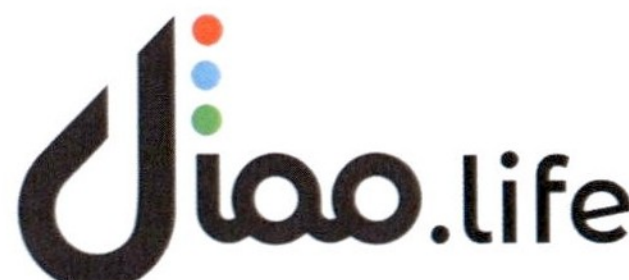

Published by Jiao Ltd

Jiao.life

Scan the QR codes to access the digital book or listen to the audio book.

Audiobook

Digital Book

The Seven Stages of Switch Development

Growing Gareth is part of the Switch Heroes, social stories created to support switch-users with their Switch progression. The Switch Heroes series is part of the Seven Stages of Switch Development, created by Occupational Therapist and AT specialist Luke Thompson.

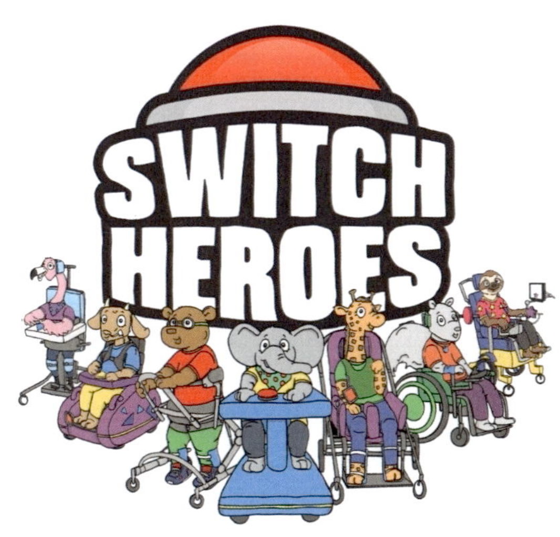

Gareth's learning switch skills

Just like you and me

What is Gareth doing?

Shall we look, and see?

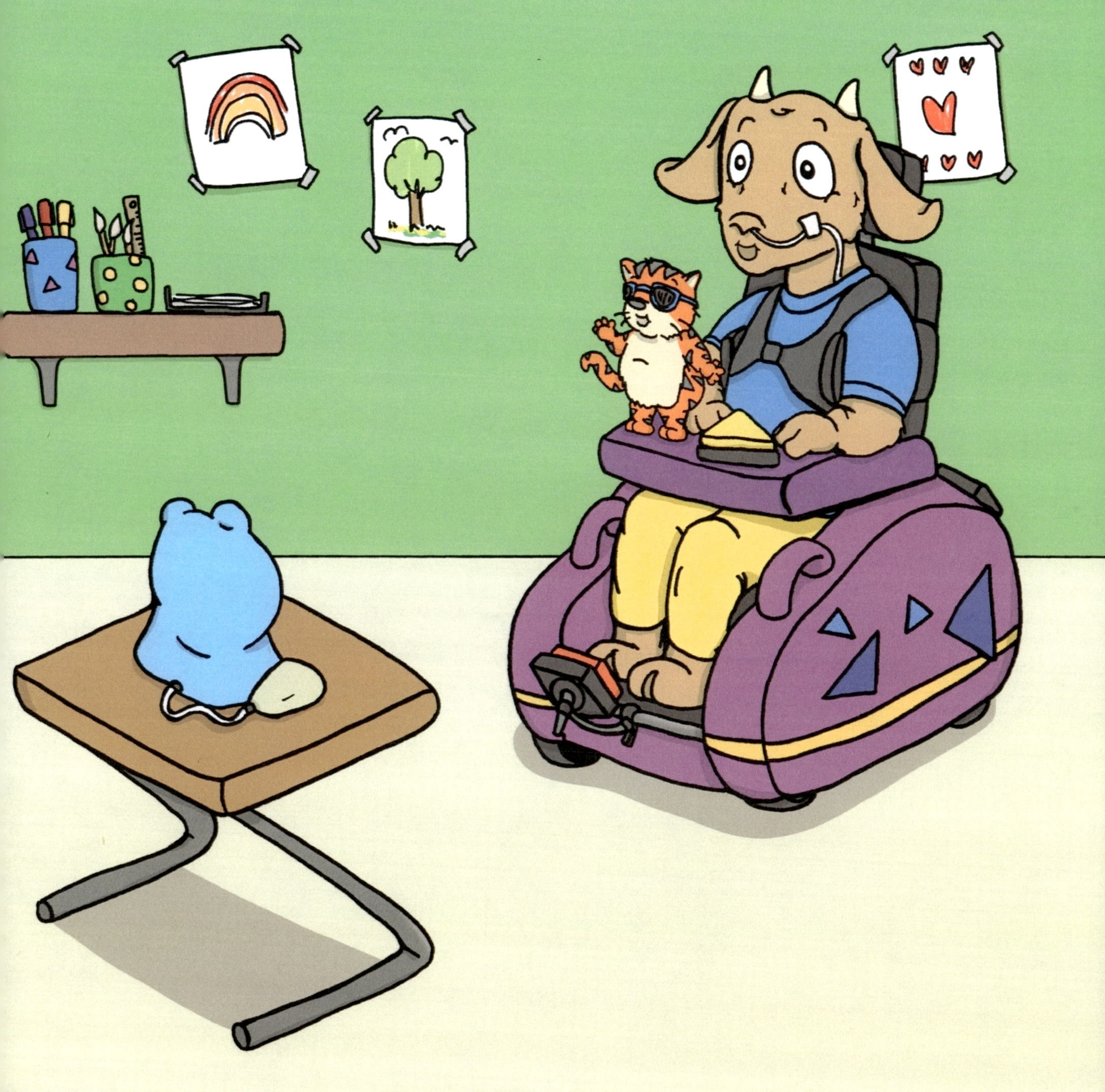

His yellow triangle button

Is plugged in over there

When he pushes down on it

Bubbles fill the air

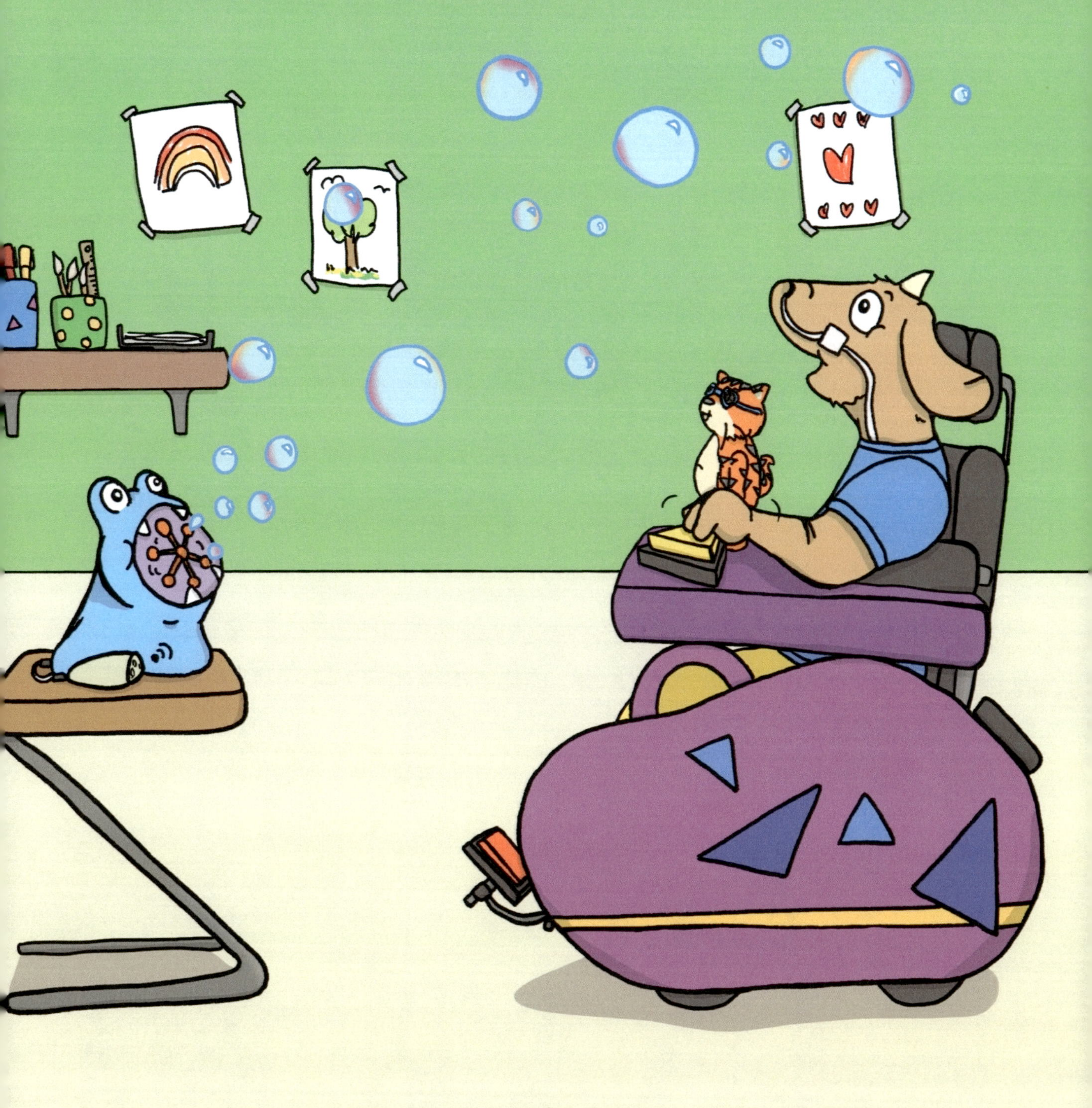

Have you got your switch here too?

Is your toy plugged in?

Demonstrate what it can do

Wow - it can dance and sing!

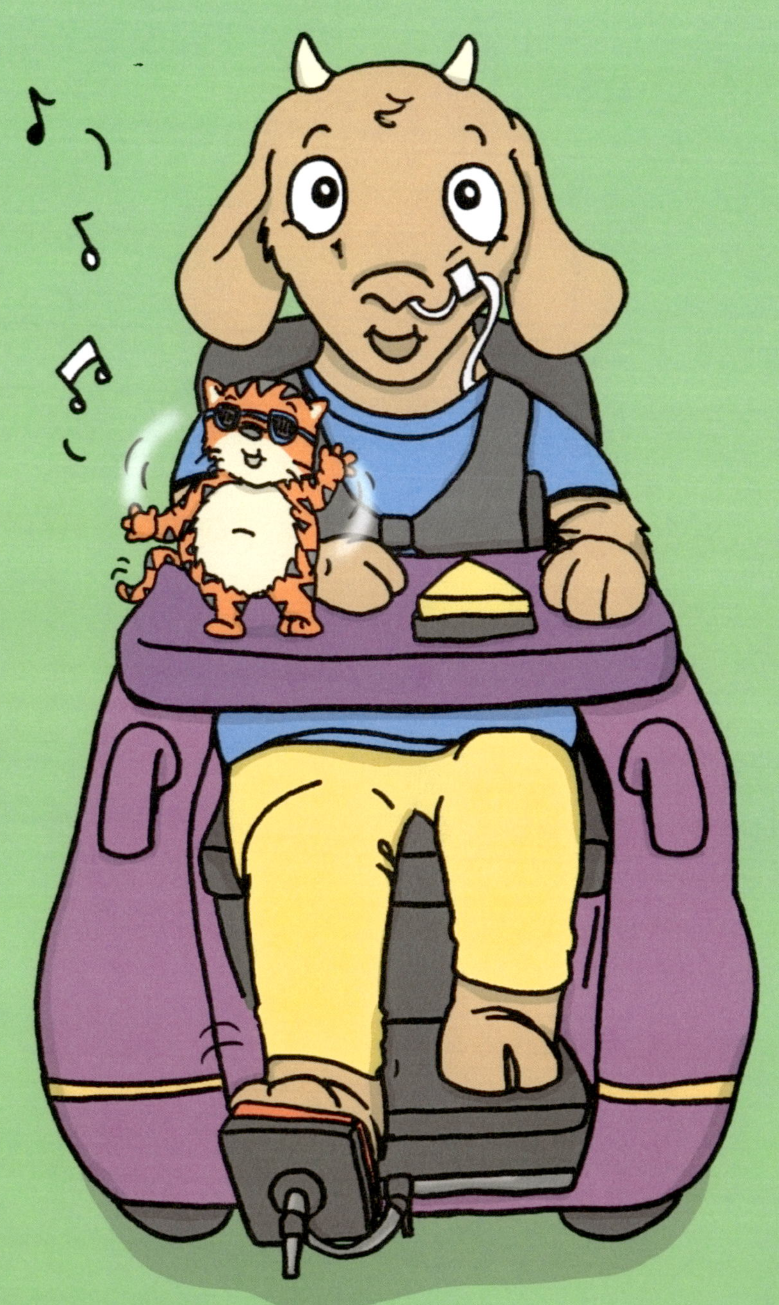

Gareth wants to show
you something

Would that be ok?

He used his switch

Now you use yours

Then both of you can play

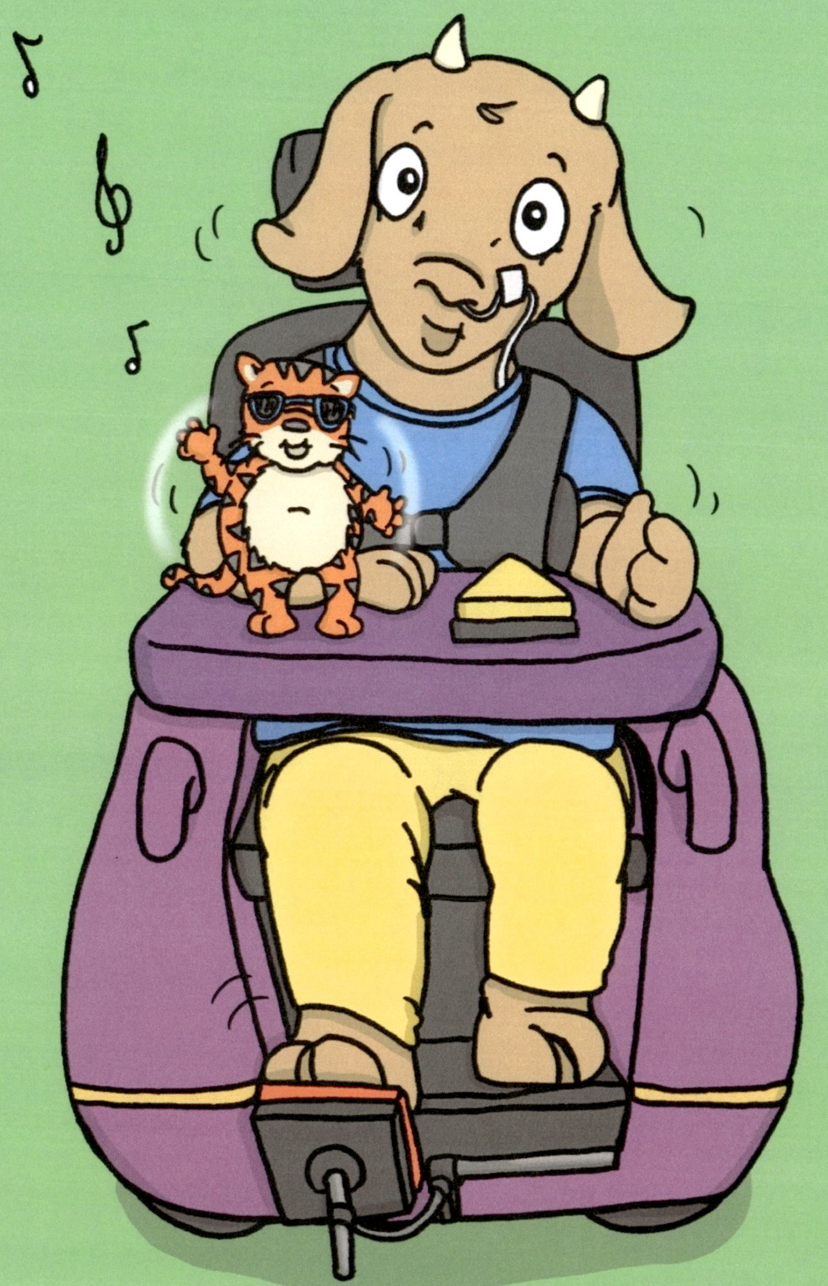

He pushes his orange switch

His toy begins to groove

He pushes the yellow one as well

The bubbles start to move

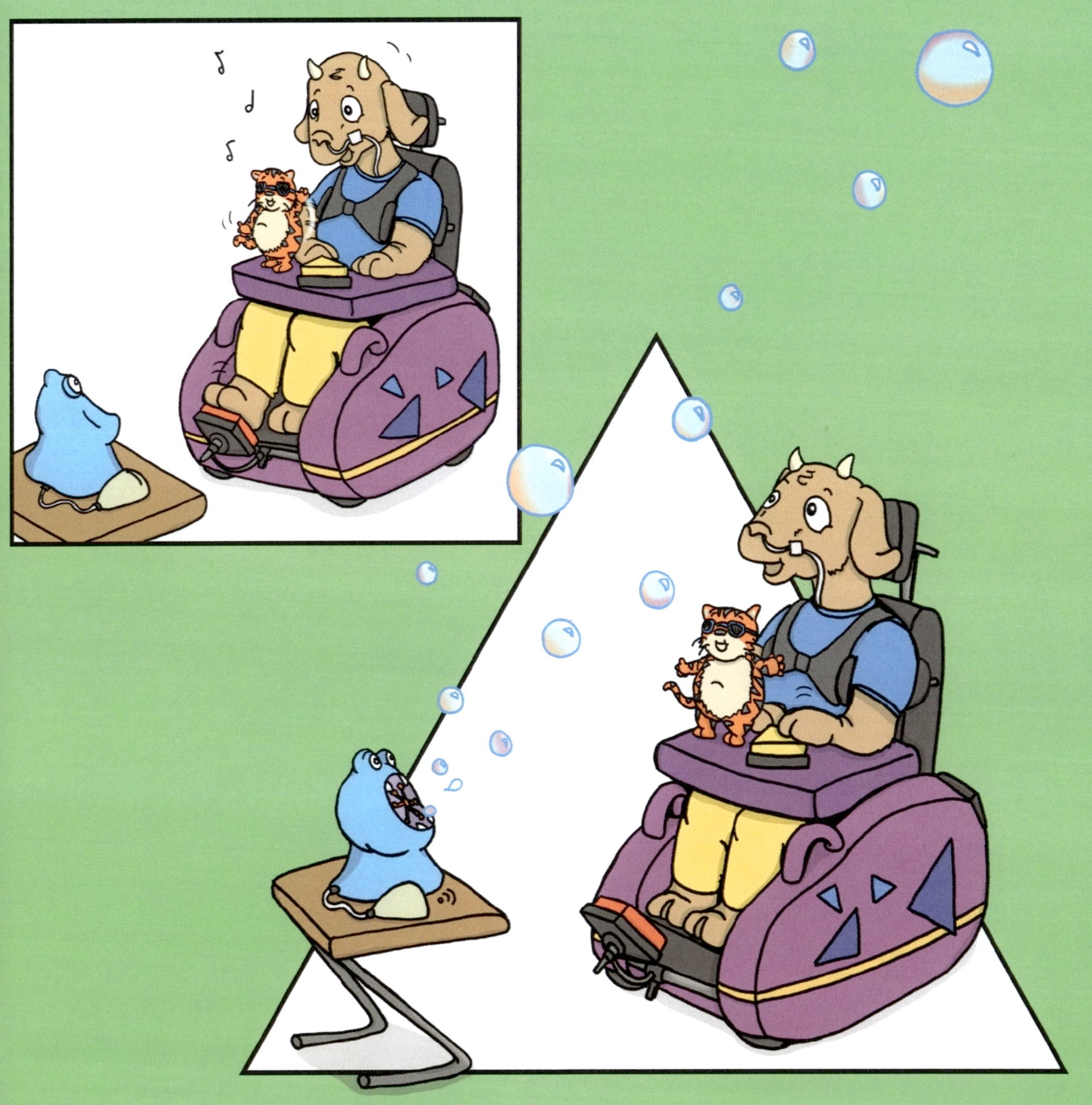

Thank you, Gareth,
for showing us

That switches are such fun

Your switch skills are developing

There's so much more to come

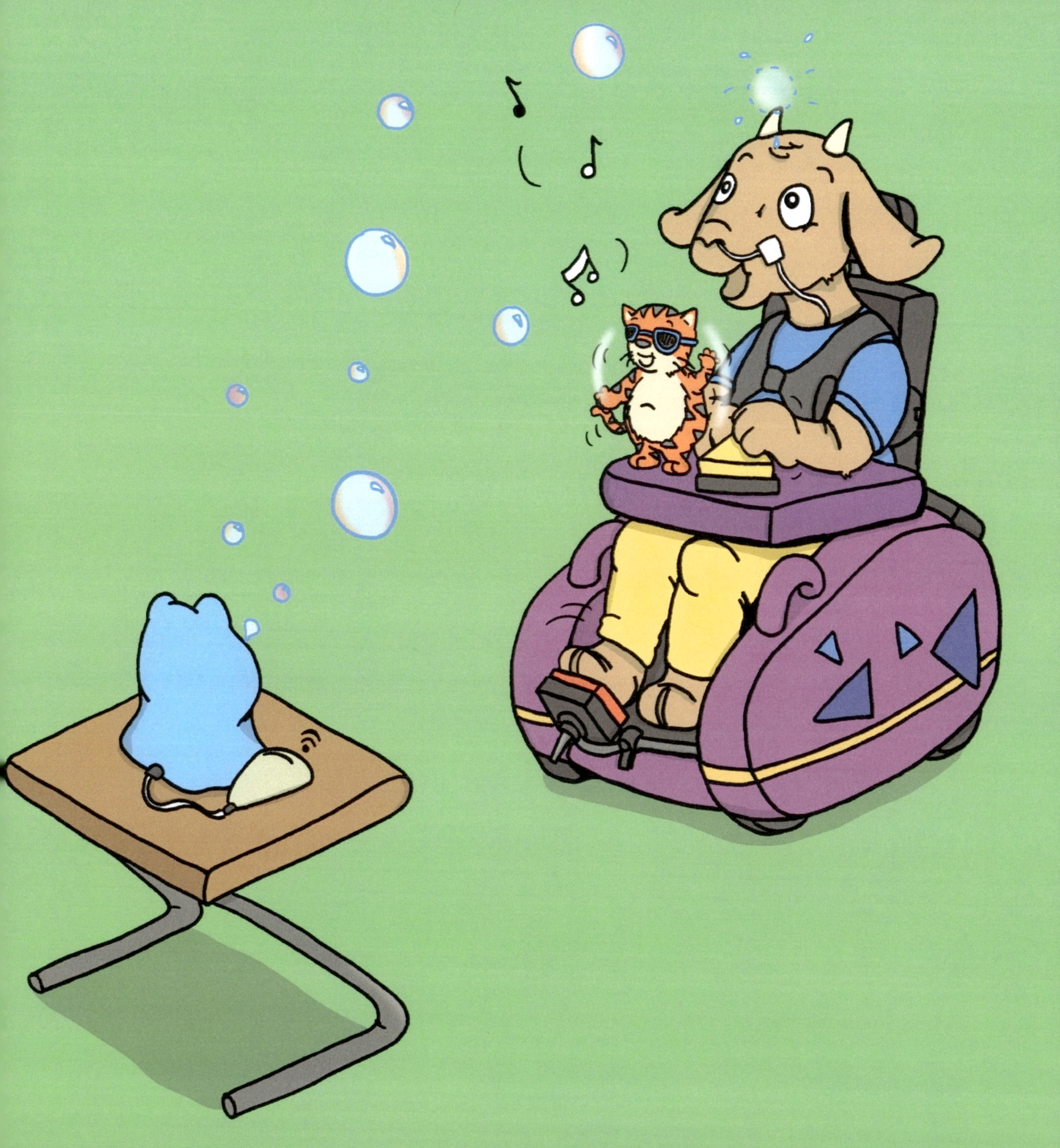

And now he's going
back and forth

Between switch one and two

Doing more than one thing

And you can do it too!

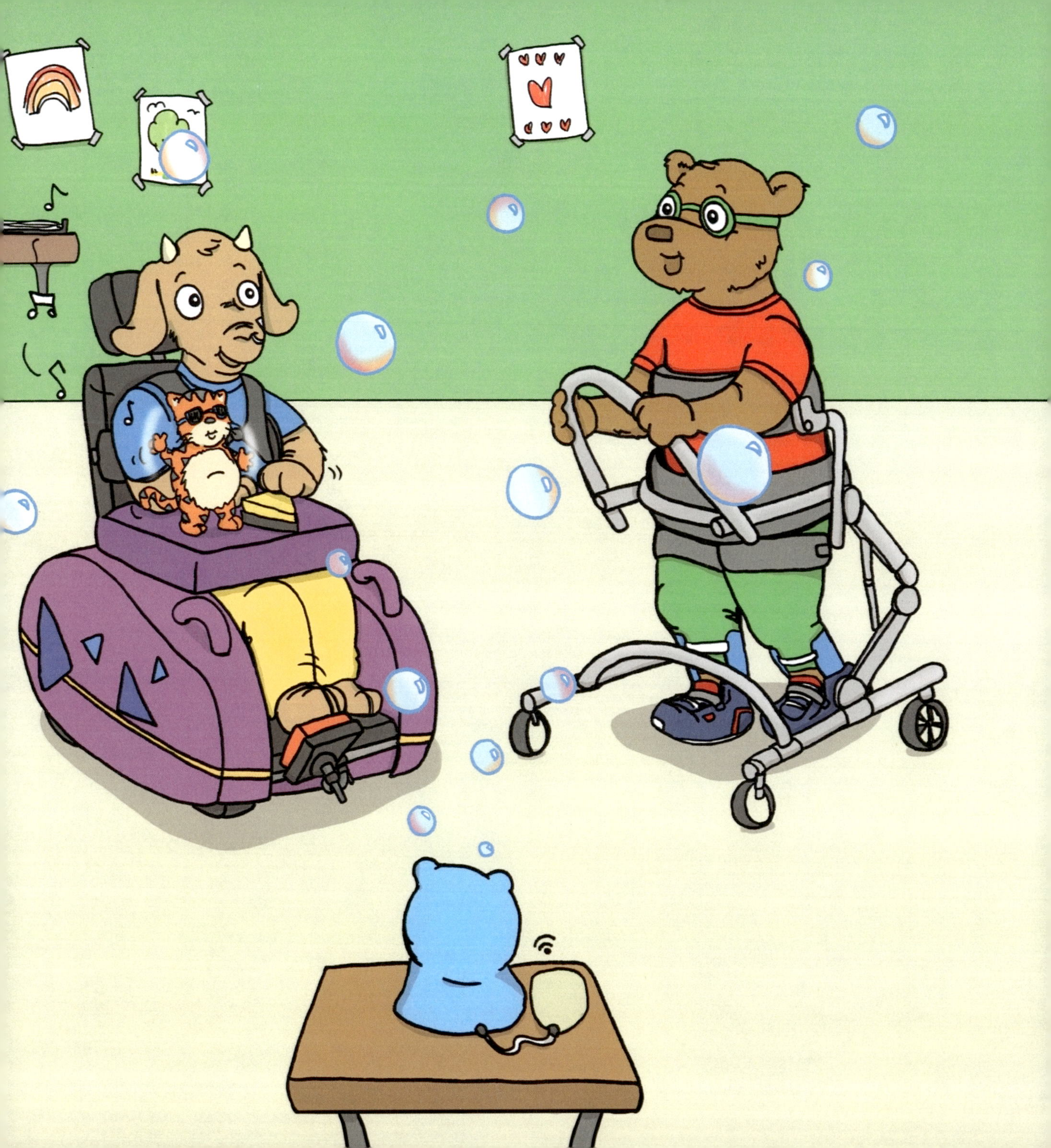

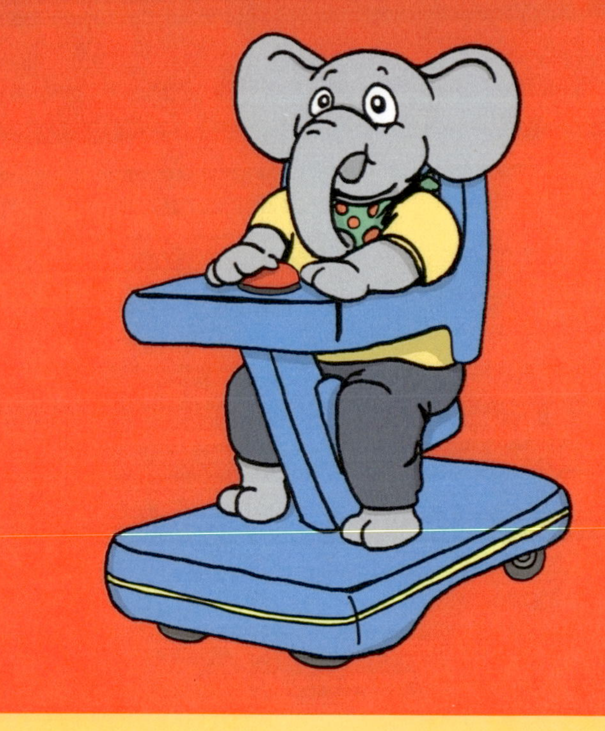
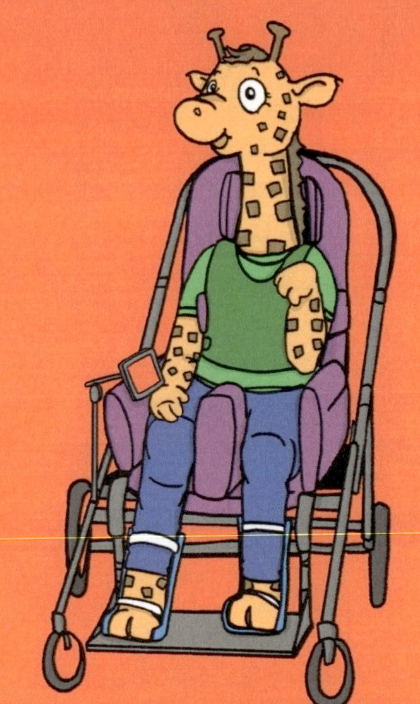
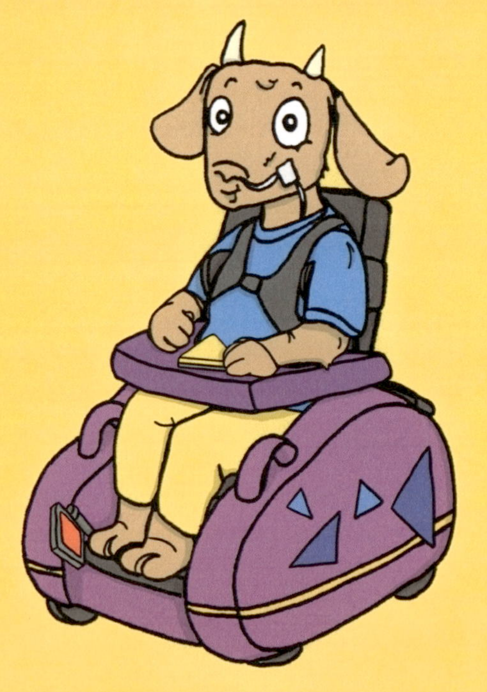
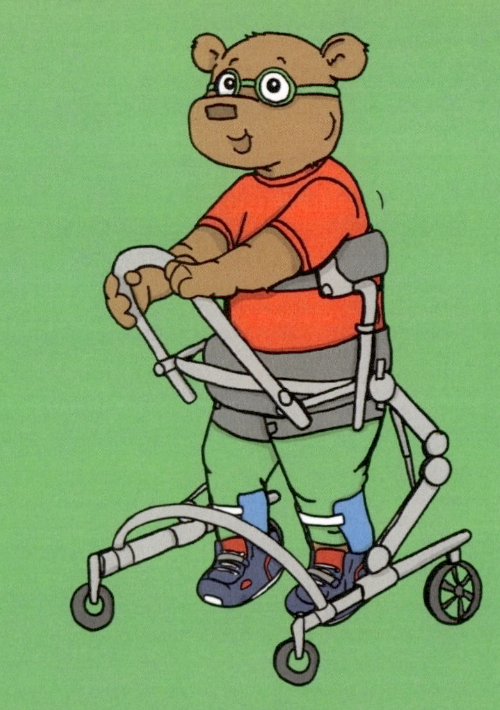

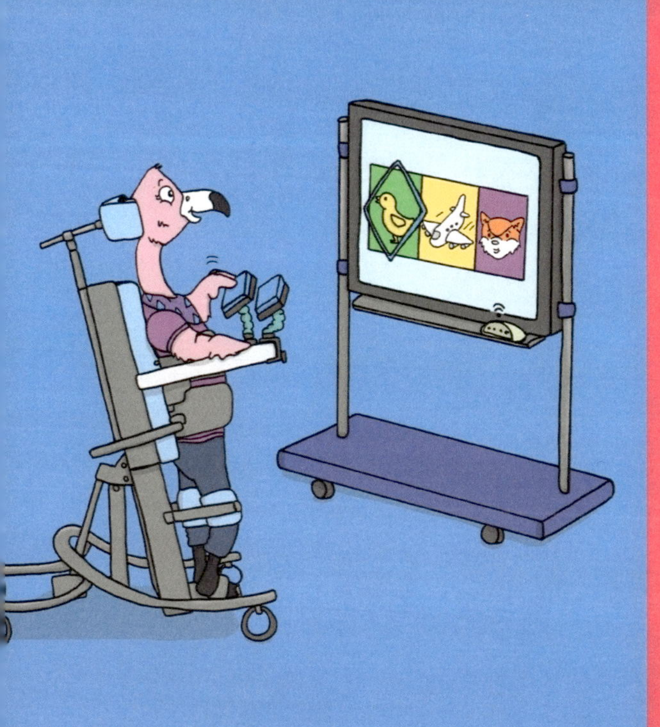

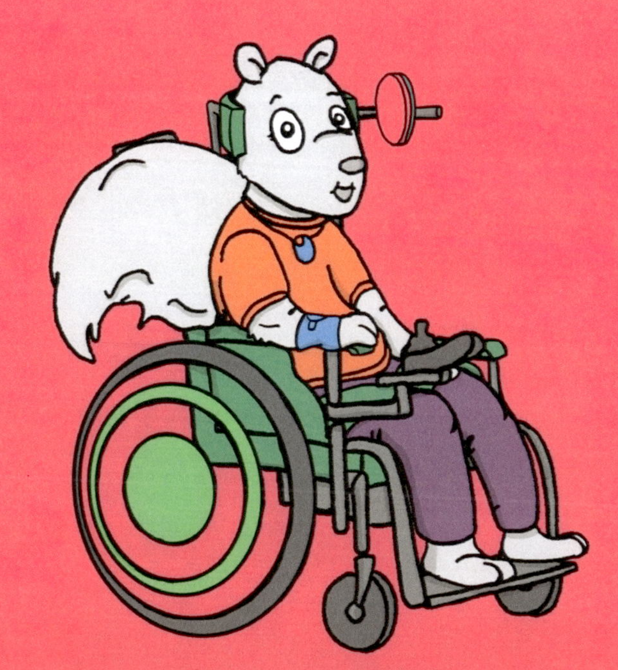

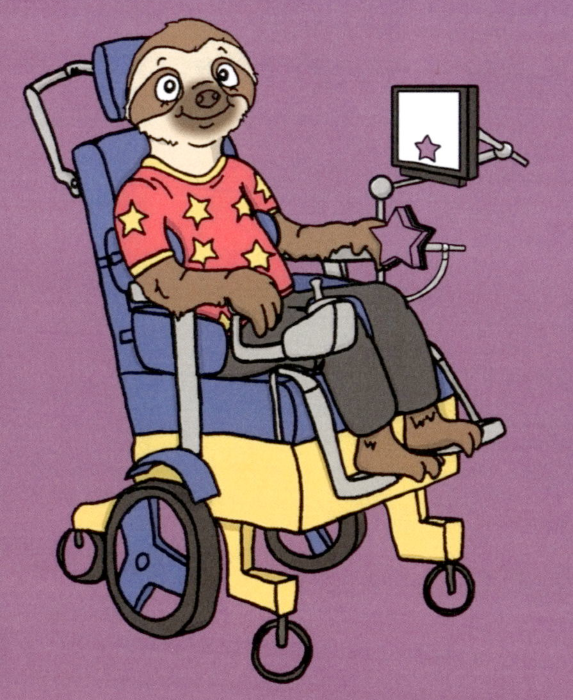

Photo of you!

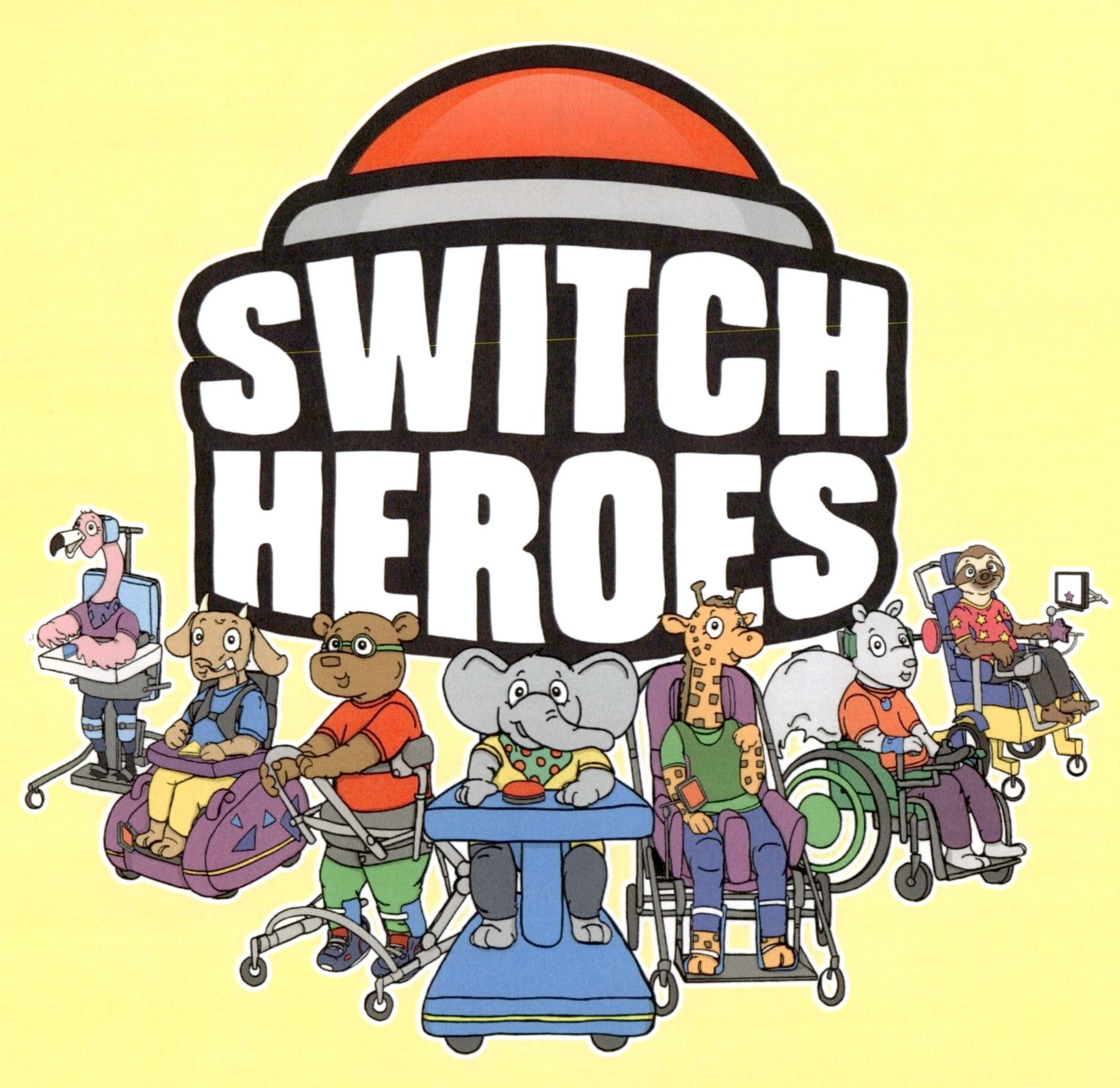

SWITCH
HEROES

The Seven Stages of Switch Development

The Seven Stages of Switch Development is a resource designed for switch-users, their families, caregivers and those who assist them in using switches. It features child-friendly characters and stories that support everyones learning.

The framework provides a helpful reference for measuring and tracking progress while offering flexibility to accommodate the unique needs and preferences of each switch-user.

Written directly to the switch-user, the framework can be read to them if they are unable to read it themselves. Our aim is to ensure that those supporting the child/switch-user can prioritise the child's needs and perspective in the process of developing their switch skills. We have seen the impact of involving the child in the learning process. Seeking their input and feedback regularly empowers them to take an active role in their development and combat learned helplessness.

Adapted from: Bean, I. (2011). Switch Progression Learning Journeys Road Map. Inclusive Technology. Burkhart, L. (2018). Stepping Stones to Switch Access. Perspectives of the ASHA Special Interest Groups, 3(12), pp.33-44. doi:https://doi/10.1044/persp3.sig12.33.

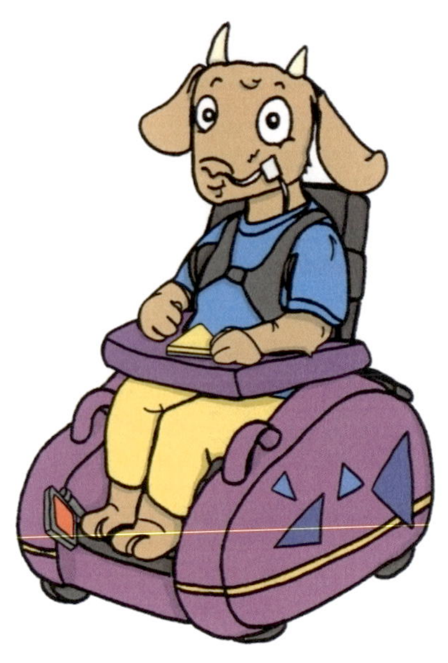

Definition

Growing Gareth is where you start to understand and use two switches to do two different things. You will have had plenty of practise with one switch, as well as using it with different parts of your body and for different activities. Now you have two switches at the same time, which are connected to two very different, simple activities.

This helps you to further understand what switches do. During this time, you can continue to have fun doing simple switch activities, but you have a new challenge of using your body to find and use two different switches that are in different places.

During this time when you play with switches, you learn about making choices. You also continue to learn what switches do and develop the physical/motor skills to use them.

- Developing understanding of two switches: You will understand that two switches can do two different things

- Primary and secondary switch sites: There will be two parts of your body that you will mainly use to activate your two switches, with lessening support or prompting from others

- You will have a good understanding of what other body parts work well or not so well when activating a switch

- Developing choice: You will show a preference between two different switch activities – pressing a preferred option more frequently and avoiding a disliked option

- Automating skills: You will have improved your motor skills, activating a switch with greater speed and efficiency

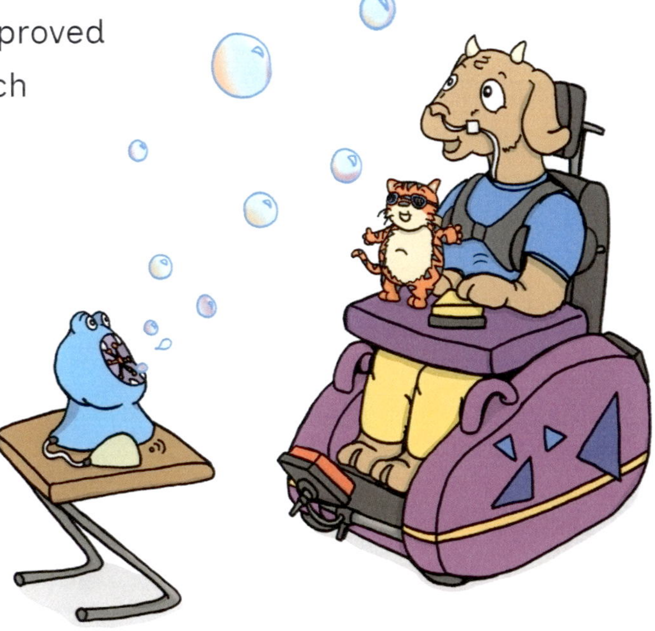

- Make sure the two switches do two very different things, one could be highly motivating, and the other might be less so (or even disliked) – swap the activities between switches to see if the activity or access is preferred

- Try not to influence the switch-user to choose a particular switch, let them explore for themselves

- Introduce the second switch in a clear, obvious and structured way – using modelling to introduce

- Provide activities that enable the switch-user to use both switches independently and together, for example, a bubble machine and a fan

- Use visual and auditory cues to help the switch-user understand the relationship between the two switches and the outcomes

- Continue building foundational skills using the easy-hard-easy principle: start with an easy task, gradually increase the difficulty, and conclude with a task that allows the user to feel successful. This approach ensures they experience a sense of accomplishment while being challenged. The child will continue to engage in single-switch activities throughout

Activities

- Try using two different switch toys; for example, one makes a switch toy move/dance/sing, and another blows a fan

- Programme two voice-output switches (or one with two-switch options) to give different commands in a fun game (e.g., 'clap your hands' and 'do a star jump')

- Computer games: there are lots of two-switch computer activities. Try simple activities that allow each switch to play a different sound or function. You can progress to more complicated two-switch activities where one switch works first and the second is redundant/plays a repeat action. Then when the steps are complete the first switch becomes redundant and the second switch finishes the activity

Instead of a prompt hierarchy where the type of prompt increase in support level, we recommend our one prompt switch support cycle. Find out more at Jiao.life

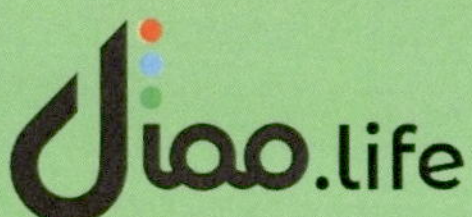

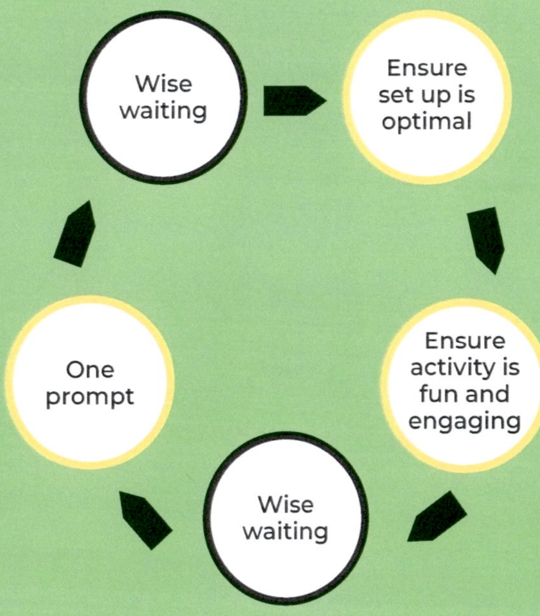

The Assessment Tool

Proficient step							
Consolidating step							
Emerging step							

Emerging – Developing – Consolidating – Proficient (cognitive, physical skill required for each stage)

Physical	E D C P	E D C P	E D C P	E D C P	E D C P	E D C P	E D C P
Cognitive	E D C P	E D C P	E D C P	E D C P	E D C P	E D C P	E D C P

The Seven Stages of Switch Development ▶

Stage 1 Exploring Egbert	Stage 2 Journeying Jiao	Stage 3 Growing Gareth	Stage 4 Budding Brayton	Stage 5 Flourishing Fatima	Stage 6 Succeeding Saffi	Stage 7 Celebrating Syed
Learning by experience – single switch	Making something happen – single switch	Playing with two switches Making two things happen	Two switches one activity	Switch scanning – failure Free	Switch scanning – finding the right one	Independent in functional switch use

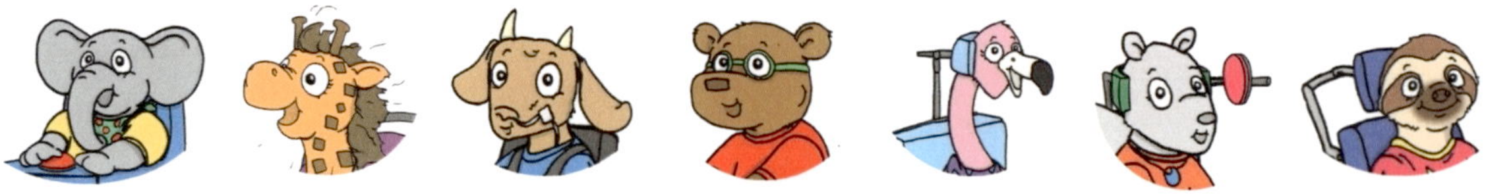

Print version available at Jiao.life

How to use the assessment tool

- The stages of switch development are not mutually exclusive, so progress can be made across multiple stages simultaneously

- Once a step is completed, mark it off and add the date

- The assessment tool can be used for goal setting, where helpers can add target dates and change the text/box colour accordingly

- There is a stream for assessing cognitive and physical skill development, divided into four steps for each stage (Emerging, Developing, Consolidating and Proficient)

- Helpers should consider the cognitive and physical skills required for each level

- This additional stream can help identify areas that may require additional support and highlight strengths and weaknesses for targeted interventions

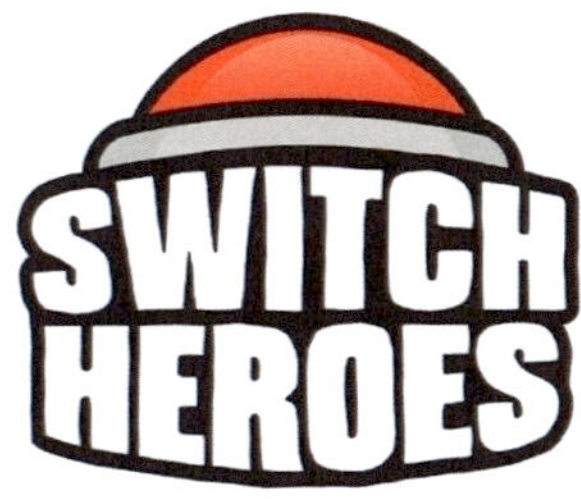

At Jiao Ltd, we are dedicated to empowering individuals through innovative assistive technology solutions.

We provide personalised services and training to help children, families, and professionals navigate the world of assistive tech. For more resources, training options, or to learn how we can support you, visit Jiao.life or get in touch with us directly. We look forward to hearing from you!

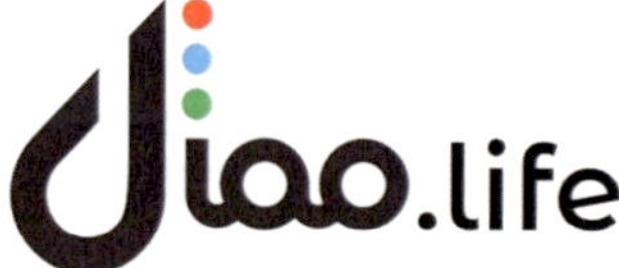

This is to certify that

____

is playing with
two switches

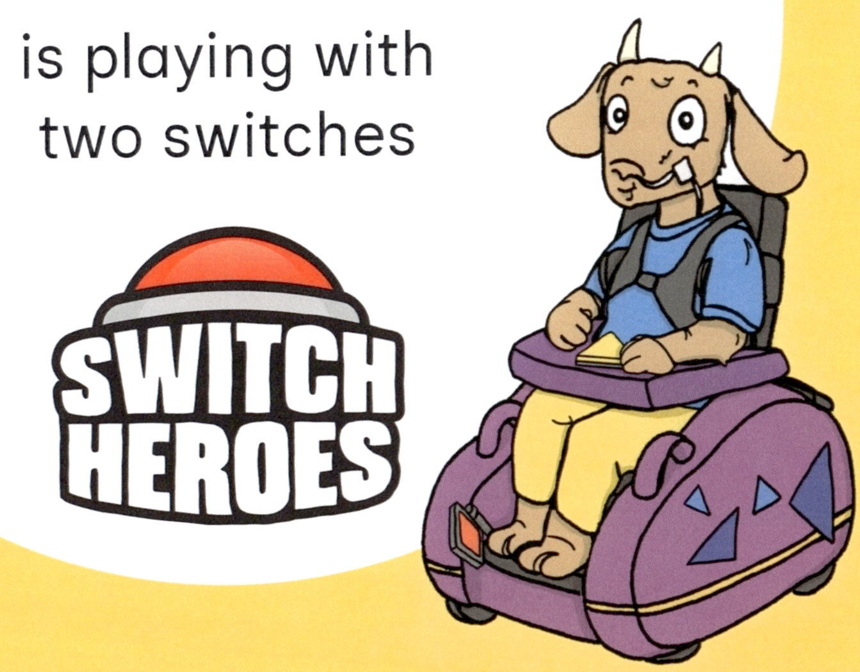